Bulletproof Diet

Reset Your Metabolism And Experience Enhanced
Energy With A Bulletproof Diet

*(A Straightforward And Delicious Guide To Kick start Your
Health)*

Normand Bourgeois

TABLE OF CONTENT

Chapter 1: Drink First When You Get Hunger Pangs

When you're feeling hungry, it's simple to go to a drive-through, the nearest restaurant, or even a corner store to purchase a ready-made meal. Indeed, you are famished. You are taking action to alleviate hunger as quickly as possible.

I understand. That is what most individuals do.

The issue is that the appetite you are experiencing may not last long. Perhaps these hunger sensations are temporary.

This is why I recommend drinking first when you feel hunger pains. You would be amazed at how rapidly your hunger disappears.

The key is to consume alcohol first. Now, don't go wild. There is no need to go above and beyond. You do not need to pull out a liter or gallon container of water and begin pounding.

No. A tiny cup would suffice. See if it solves the problem. Then, drink another glass.

Another strategy I employ is to first consume tepid water. If available, consume a small amount of lukewarm water. You would be astonished at how many of your hunger pangs are actually your body's attempt to rehydrate itself.

Follow this plan: when you experience hunger pains, drink warm water first, followed by cold water. If that doesn't work, you should decide to consume.

Chew Slowly

Once you've decided to consume, take your time with the process. I recognize that this is simpler said than done.

If you are like the majority of Americans, you feel like you don't have much time. If you are like most people, you would consider time a luxury. Believe me, I completely understand where you're coming from and your position.

However, here's the deal. If you rush through your meal, your brain will not register complete satiety. It will remain partially famished.

So, what do you anticipate will occur next? That is correct. You consume additional calories until you are ultimately satisfied. Typically, in this context, the body only feels filled when the stomach has sufficiently expanded.

As you can assume, this is not a weight loss recipe. You wind up eating excessively. This is why eating carefully is recommended.

You are consuming ketogenic dishes. That is amazing. However, eat carefully.

This allows you to appreciate your sustenance more. It also allows the brain to synchronize and align with the body.

Because when you consume, chemical compounds are released throughout your body. It is transmitting a variety of signals. There is interaction between the brain and the remainder of the body, especially the digestive tract.

This delicate balance of signals cascading into each other and reacting is not completely realized if you rush through your meals. Therefore, you overwhelm your system with calories.

Chew carefully. There is no hurry. Savor every morsel. Celebrate your cuisine.

Again, food is necessary for survival. Don't eat to survive.

Eliminate Milk-Based Snacks Gradually.

For many individuals, milk is a sensitive topic. Many individuals on a ketogenic diet can do without cola. Many individuals can acclimate to a diet of grain-free snacks with relative ease. The issue is that they become agitated when attempting to eliminate milk and dairy-based products.

I therefore recommend a gradual reduction. I don't mean permanently, and I don't want to undergo a rapid withdrawal process; I simply intend to reduce my consumption of milk-based snacks and meals gradually.

The key is to pace yourself in accordance with your evolving preferences. You should in no way accelerate this procedure.

Remember the aforementioned guidelines for meal planning. Ensure that you attempt them all. If you are experiencing trouble with one, keep trying.

There is no need to portray the hero once more. There is no need for a solitary, tremendous leap. You are making no endeavor to convince anyone of anything.

In this situation, it is crucial that you can maintain the changes you've made. Small, incremental adjustments can have significant effects.

Some individuals are extremely adaptable. Some people require a little more effort. Determine which one you are, then implement the strategy.

Your body will adapt to it eventually. Your taste receptors will change over time.

Chapter 2: Drink First When You Get Hunger Pangs

When you're feeling hungry, it's simple to go to a drive-through, the nearest restaurant, or even a corner store to purchase a ready-made meal. Indeed, you are famished. You are taking action to alleviate hunger as quickly as possible.

I understand. That is what most individuals do.

The issue is that the appetite you are experiencing may not last long. Perhaps these hunger sensations are temporary.

This is why I recommend drinking first when you feel hunger pains. You would be amazed at how rapidly your hunger disappears.

The key is to consume alcohol first. Now, don't go wild. There is no need to go above and beyond. You do not need to pull out a liter or gallon container of water and begin pounding.

No. A tiny cup would suffice. See if it solves the problem. Then, drink another glass.

Another strategy I employ is to first consume tepid water. If available, consume a small amount of lukewarm water. You would be astonished at how many of your hunger pangs are actually your body's attempt to rehydrate itself.

Follow this plan: when you experience hunger pains, drink warm water first, followed by cold water. If that doesn't work, you should decide to consume.

Chew Slowly

Once you've decided to consume, take your time with the process. I recognize that this is simpler said than done.

If you are like the majority of Americans, you feel like you don't have much time. If you are like most people, you would consider time a luxury. Believe me, I completely understand where you're coming from and your position.

However, here's the deal. If you rush through your meal, your brain will not register complete satiety.

It will remain partially famished.

So, what do you anticipate will occur next? That is correct. You consume additional calories until you are ultimately satisfied.

Typically, in this context, the body only feels filled when the stomach has sufficiently expanded.

As you can assume, this is not a weight loss recipe. You wind up eating excessively. This is why eating carefully is recommended.

You are consuming ketogenic dishes. That is amazing. However, eat carefully.

This allows you to appreciate your sustenance more. It also allows the brain to synchronize and align with the body.

Because when you consume, chemical compounds are released throughout your body. It is transmitting a variety of signals. There is interaction between the brain and the remainder of the body, especially the digestive tract.

This delicate balance of signals cascading into each other and reacting is not completely realized if you rush through your meals. Therefore, you overwhelm your system with calories.

Chew carefully. There is no hurry. Savor every morsel. Celebrate your cuisine.

Again, food is necessary for survival. Don't eat to survive.

Circadian Rhythm

Restorative sleep is essential for CFS recovery. As a result of their interference with our circadian rhythm, modern life is rife with factors that impede restful slumber. Circadian rhythm is fundamentally each individual's internal clock. It regulates the secretion of hormones, stomach acid, pancreatic enzymes, and other substances. Moreover, when your circadian rhythm is trained to a consistent sleep schedule, you enjoy heavenly, restful slumber.

There are distinct stages of slumber that a person enters at various times during sleep. Stages 2 and 2 are dreaming states of light slumber during which the body does not heal. Stages 6 and 8 are much deeper states in which the body repairs and restores itself. Life in the twenty-first century makes it more difficult to enter these deeper phases of sleep. Our circadian rhythm is affected by the amount of light we are exposed to throughout the day. The most prominent cause of imbalance is exposure to blue light. Televisions, computers, phones, and other indoor lights stimulate the eyes' receptors and fool the brain into believing it is still daytime. As damaging is the dearth of natural sunlight during the day, which is caused by the requirement that people work and live indoors.

How do we therefore retrain our circadian rhythm? You must adhere to strict guidelines regarding your exposure to light. Turn off all electronic devices one hour before bedtime, or even better, two hours! Instead of using your phone, try reading a book, playing a board game, keeping a journal, meditating, or conversing with your family. It may take some time to retrain your brain so you are no longer compelled to reach for your phone, but you will be so happy you made the effort. If you must use your electronic devices at night, use glasses that block blue light and mild light settings.

Upon awakening, the next phase is to obtain as much light as possible. Go outside and gaze at the heavens, avoiding the sun but exposing your eyes to light. If the weather is cloudy where you reside, you can purchase a clip-on blue light that shines directly into your eye. The Feel Bright Light is utilized. It attaches to any baseball cap, and I appreciate that I can do other things while it helps me wake up in the morning. Before 2 0 a.m., it is essential to receive at least 6 0 minutes of bright light above 2 0,000 lux. Regularly performing this will assist in regulating your cortisol arousal cycle and all of your feel-good hormones.

But most importantly, harmonizing your circadian rhythm will improve your digestion, regulate your autonomic nervous system, enhance your sleep, and promote cellular healing.

Chapter 3: Here Are Some General Recommendations For Your Meals.

Fruit and starch should only account for 10 % of your daily caloric intake. If losing weight is your top priority. Try to avoid them as much as possible. If not, you may consume a modest portion daily.

20% of your calories should come from vegetables without carbohydrates. Because vegetables are low in calories, they will occupy a significant portion of your plate. If you dislike vegetables, you can coat them in grass-fed butter and sea salt.

Protein sources should be indestructible and comprise 20% of your caloric intake.

100 to 70 percent of a person's daily calorie consumption should consist of healthy fats.

If you're not hungry, don't force yourself to consume. If you do not adhere to the daily recommendations, it is not a huge deal.

When famished, consume food. Stop eating when satiated. If possible, avoid snacking as much as possible.

Breakfast

Consume two glasses of piping hot Bulletproof coffee. Use exclusively Bulletproof Upgraded Coffee. These beans are of the utmost quality and contain no mold or toxins. Add 2 teaspoons of butter. Ensure that the butter is from grass-fed cows and unsalted. Two tablespoons of Brain Octane C8 Medium Chain Triglyceride Oil or any other MCT oil may also be added. If you have no other options, coconut oil can be used. You could also add powdered cinnamon, chocolate, or vanilla of the utmost quality. Use xylitol, erythritol, or stevia according to flavor.

If you need to lose a significant amount of weight, are a heavily muscled athlete, or are a woman, you should consume some form of protein with your Bulletproof Coffee for the first sixty days. Collagen protein derived from grass-fed poultry is recommended for use in Bulletproof coffee.

If you are pregnant or attempting to conceive, you should avoid drinking caffeinated coffee. Try the recipe for No-

Coffee Vanilla Latte (located in the chapter on Breakfast Recipes) or use lab-tested decaf.

After fourteen days, or what we refer to as maintenance mode, you can consume something other than Bulletproof Coffee. A combination of oil and protein, such as avocado, smoked salmon, and a poached egg, is optimal. Although consuming protein without fat is preferable to consuming carbohydrates or fruits, you may still experience cravings.

Intermittent Fasting

Do not consume anything after your morning coffee until lunch, or later if you are not famished. This allows you to reap the benefits of intermittent fasting while still eating breakfast.

Your dietary window lasts six hours. This results in a fast of 2 8 hours.

Evening Meal

Consume a sufficient quantity of Bulletproof carbohydrates. This should include approximately 6 0 grams of vegetables. Consume only with your evening supper. Have a carb refeed day once or twice per week. On these days, consume between 2 00 and 2 100 grams. This should be performed on days when you are Bulletproof Protein fasting. How rapidly you want to lose weight, your stress level, and your hunger will determine the quantity. Consuming fewer carbohydrates every night will expedite weight loss.

On refeed days, women need at least 6 00 grams more carbohydrates. If you are expectant, you should limit your carbohydrate intake at night while adhering to all other Bulletproof Diet principles.

Indulge in fat at supper. This improves your slumber. Additionally, adding protein before bedtime can aid in sleep. Avoid eating too much flesh. This can leave you feeling burdened. Utilize undenatured whey protein concentrate or grass-fed collagen peptide that has been hydrolyzed. Additionally, you could consume organic honey. These may also be added to the No-Coffee Vanilla Latte.

Rapid Protein Digestion

Once per week, consume a maximum of 210 grams of protein.

If you discover that protein deprivation causes muscle loss or other adverse effects, you can reduce your intake. Instead of skipping protein for an entire day, avoid it for a few meals. On Bulletproof Protein Fasting days, you are free to experiment with the amount of protein you consume.

Protocol Bulletproof for two weeks

Get rid of all the unhealthy snack food in your home.

Utilize as a guide the food guidance from the previous chapter. Focus on the Good foods and avoid the test foods and poor ingredients as much as possible.

Bulletproof coffee should be consumed for morning. If you need to lose a significant amount of weight, are a woman over the age of 8 0, or if coffee does not satisfy your hunger, you can add 210 to 6 0 grams of protein, such as grass-fed collagen protein.

You must consume enormous quantities of vegetables for lunch and supper. Additionally, consume healthy lipids, a moderate amount of protein, and a small amount of carbohydrates after and during dinner. Consume both meals within a six-hour interval for intermittent fasting to be effective. For instance, have lunch at 2 p.m. and supper at 7 p.m.

Once per week, typically on days 6 and 2 6 , adhere to the Bulletproof Protein

Fasting. This necessitates the consumption of 210 grams of protein and 2 00 to 2 100 grams of carbohydrates. If you are a woman, you are permitted to consume 6 00 grams of carbohydrates.

Make sure you maintain track of the unhealthy foods you've identified. Each individual has unique culinary sensitivities.

If you suspect dietary allergies, your doctor can perform a blood panel test.

Start this testing during the two-week protocol to determine if any specific healthy foods are actually unhealthy for you.

This document contains a shopping list that may facilitate your journey to the grocery store. Obviously, you do not need to acquire everything. Its sole purpose is to provide options. You can select from the available options in your area.

Chapter 4: Inflammation In The Human Body's Causes

Lectins are specialized forms of proteins produced by plants to protect themselves from predators, such as us. There are tens of thousands of lectins, and they attach themselves irreversibly to the carbohydrates that line the cells of your body; as a result, they may interfere with cell metabolism. There are lectins that cause significant damage to the cells of the small intestine and the gut villi, which are tiny projections on the inner walls of the small intestine that aid in the absorption of nutrients from the foods you consume. Some of the harmful lectins produced by plants can irritate the gut, bond to the joints, cause bacterial overgrowth in the intestines, and even cause Leptin resistance. Leptin is one of the hormones that helps convey to the brain when you are full, so it has a direct effect on your appetite. Leptin resistance occurs when the brain loses sensitivity to the hormonal signals from Leptin, leading to an out-of-control appetite and a multitude of other diseases.

Lectins are present in numerous food types. However, certain foods, such as cereals, nuts, and legumes, contain a high concentration of lectins. Therefore, the more of these foods you ingest, the greater the likelihood that the lectins in these foods will cause an allergic reaction in various parts of your body, leading to inflammation.

Not everyone will have the same allergic reaction to various types of lectins; some people will be more sensitive than others to the lectins found in certain types of foods. Migraines, poor skin, achy joints, and brain fog are among the initial symptoms of lectin-induced allergic reactions. Many individuals are sensitive to the lectins found in nightshade plants (such as potatoes, peppers, eggplants, and tomatoes) and will experience allergic reactions if they consume these plants. In fact, these plants have been linked to a substantial proportion of cases of skin disorders and rheumatoid arthritis.

The good news is that the majority of lectins are destroyed by heat, so they can be reduced or eliminated from foods by employing specific cooking techniques. Additionally, you can avoid all foods that contain large quantities of allergenic lectins. This is what the bulletproof diet is all about: educating you on the harmful substances in foods that cause allergic reactions in your body and encouraging you to avoid these foods and substitute them with healthier alternatives.

Phytates are also substances produced by plants to discourage insect and animal consumption. They accomplish this by binding to the essential minerals in our nutrition, such as calcium, magnesium, zinc, and iron. When they bind in this manner to our dietary minerals, their absorption is slowed or prevented entirely. As you can imagine, consuming these plants on a regular basis would cause deficiency diseases in both animals and humans, and we would soon realize that they are the cause of the problems and cease consuming them. In the wild, animals quickly learn to avoid these phytate-containing plants, whereas humans have become so dependent on phytate-rich seeds, nuts, and whole cereals that we continue to consume them. Worse still, the majority of us have not even considered that phytate-producing plants are primarily responsible for our deficiencies in certain nutrients and minerals.

Even phytates are antioxidants, which is why these foods are often labeled as high in antioxidants (substances that prevent other molecules from being damaged or oxidized). However, not all antioxidants are the same, and some, such as phytates, can cause harm to the body. It will be difficult to completely eliminate phytates from your diet, but you can make dietary changes to reduce the amount of high-phytate foods you ingest and you can also modify your cooking techniques to reduce the amount of phytates in your food. To reduce the amount of phytates in certain high-phytate foods, you can cook them and then discard the cooking water, or you can marinate them in something acidic, such as vinegar or lemon juice. Certain seeds and cereals contain phytates that cannot be eliminated by the methods described above, so you should avoid them entirely.

Certain animals, such as sheep and cows, contain microorganisms in their digestive tracts that are capable of degrading phytates. We lack these bacteria, but when we consume grass-fed sheep and cattle that have not been fed other hazardous manufactured products, they filter out the harmful phytates for us, allowing us to absorb the other beneficial chemicals in these foods without the harmful phytates.

Chapter 5: Drink First When You Get Hunger Pangs

When you're feeling hungry, it's simple to go to a drive-through, the nearest restaurant, or even a corner store to purchase a ready-made meal. Indeed, you are famished. You are taking action to alleviate hunger as quickly as possible.

I understand. That is what most individuals do.

The issue is that the appetite you are experiencing may not last long. Perhaps these hunger sensations are temporary.

This is why I recommend drinking first when you feel hunger pains. You would be amazed at how rapidly your hunger disappears.

The key is to consume alcohol first. Now, don't go wild. There is no need to go above and beyond. You do not need to pull out a liter or gallon container of water and begin pounding.

No. A tiny cup would suffice. See if it solves the problem. Then, drink another glass.

Another strategy I employ is to first consume tepid water. If available, consume a small amount of lukewarm water. You would be astonished at how many of your hunger pangs are actually your body's attempt to rehydrate itself.

When experiencing hunger pains, warm water should be consumed first, followed by cold water. If that doesn't work, you should decide to consume.

Once you've decided to consume, take your time with the process. I recognize that this is simpler said than done.

If you are like the majority of Americans, you feel like you don't have much time. If you are like most people, you would consider time a luxury. Believe me, I completely understand where you're coming from and your position.

However, here's the deal. If you rush through your meal, your brain will not register complete satiety. It will remain partially famished.

So, what do you anticipate will occur next? That is correct. You consume additional calories until you are ultimately satisfied. Typically, in this context, the body only feels filled when the stomach has sufficiently expanded.

As you can assume, this is not a weight loss recipe. You wind up eating excessively. This is why eating carefully is recommended.

You are consuming ketogenic dishes. That is amazing. However, eat carefully.

This allows you to appreciate your sustenance more. It also allows the brain to synchronize and align with the body.

Because when you consume, chemical compounds are released throughout your body. It is transmitting a variety of signals. There is interaction between the brain and the remainder of the body, especially the digestive tract.

This delicate balance of signals cascading into each other and reacting is not completely realized if you rush through your meals. Therefore, you overwhelm your system with calories.

Chew carefully. There is no hurry. Savor every morsel. Celebrate your cuisine.

Again, food is necessary for survival. Don't eat to survive.

Coffee Frappuccino Smoothie With Bulletproof Coffee

Ingredients

1-5 teaspoon of salt

6 tablespoons of raw honey

4 cups of almond milk, or of choice

1 teaspoon of raw organic milk

4 teaspoons of Bulletproof Coffee, or of choice

Directions

Freeze all of the ingredients after combining them in a plastic container. Remove the container from the freezer and thaw it until it is only slightly chilled and pliable enough to be processed by the blender. Pour the refrigerated soft mixture into a blender and process until smooth.

How To Make Chili With Meat

List of Ingredients

160 Grams of chili

100 Grams of hot pepper

240 Grams of tomato

160 Ml of stock

450 Grams of kidney beans

100 Grams of onion

100 Grams of garlic

1000 Grams of beef

1. To begin, fry the onion and garlic until they are golden-yellow in color.

2. After the onion and garlic have been cooked, add the sirloin and cook for a few minutes over high heat.
3. Once the beef has been browned, add the chili and seasonings and reduce the heat.
4. Now, stir in the chilies, tomatoes, and stock.
5. After adding these ingredients, simmer the sauce for 10 to 15 minutes until it has reduced. Finally, add the kidney beans 10 to 15 minutes prior to the end to ensure that they are thoroughly heated.
6. The dish can then be garnished with a swirl of fat-free fromage frais and minced herbs and paprika.
7. This dish can be served on a large jacket potato with an abundance of rice.

Similarities In The Ketogenic And Atkins Diets

Both the Atkins and keto diets involve carbohydrate restriction, and the results may be comparable.

Weight decrease

For weight loss, many individuals follow the keto or Atkins diets. Numerous studies have demonstrated that these diets can result in weight loss because the body consumes fat very efficiently when it enters ketosis. Most relevant studies indicate that a low-carb diet results in greater short-term weight loss than a low-fat diet, but both diets produce similar long-term weight loss.

A small-scale study examined Diabetes & Metabolic Syndrome: Clinical Research and Reviews indicate that ketosis may aid in the management of obesity and metabolic syndrome, both of which are risk factors for type 2 diabetes. However, confirming these findings will necessitate additional research.

Potential health advantages

A study published in the European Journal of Clinical Nutrition suggests that ketogenic diets protect the body from certain diseases, including type 2 diabetes and cardiovascular disease.

These benefits may result from a reduction in highly refined, high-sugar foods and added sugar.

Emerging evidence suggests that these diets may help with other conditions, such as Alzheimer's disease and neurological disorders, although verifying this will require additional research.

Fosu on organic cuisine

Both diets promote the consumption of unprocessed foods. Highly refined foods are associated with obesity, sardinosis, and other health conditions.

Blend Of Fennel And Carrot

Ingredients:

2 cup water

2 tablespoon lemon juice

2 small fennel bulb, sliced

4 carrots, sliced

4 pineapple slices

Directions:

1. Mix all the ingredients in a powerful blender or food processor and pulse until smooth and creamy.
2. Pour the drink in glasses and serve it as fresh as possible.

Super Green Smoothie

Ingredients:

1/2   cup cilantro

2 lemon, juiced

2 cup coconut water

4 cups baby spinach

2 cucumber, sliced

2 avocado, peeled and pitted

2 celery stalk

Directions:

Steam the spinach for 10 to 15 minutes before transferring it to a blender.

In a blender, combine the cucumber, avocado, celery, cilantro, lemon juice, and water.

Blend until smooth and creamy, then pour into glasses and serve as soon as feasible.

Bulletproof Coffee-Flavoured Ice Cream

Ingredients:

- 2 tbsp unsweetened cocoa powder
- 2 cup freshly brewed coffee
- 4 tbsp swerve sugar
- 1 cup ice

- 8 whole fresh eggs
- 8 yolks
- 2 lime, juice
- 4 tsp vanilla extract
- 2 tbsp MCT oil
- 2 tbsp unsalted butter

1. Mix all the ingredients in a blender and transfer to an ice cream maker.
2. Churn according to the manufacturer's instructions. Pour into a loaf tin, chill for 1-5 hours and enjoy after.

Adaptogenic Bulletproof Coffee

Ingredients:

- 2 tsp MCT oil
- 2 tsp coconut oil

- 2 cup freshly brewed herbal coffee
- 2 tsp heavy cream

Instructions:

Mix all the ingredients in a blender and fill in a glass.

Salad Of Chicken With Coconut Vinaigrette

4 tsp. to s. grated coconut

80 g sprouted seeds

4 avocados

the juice of 4 limes

2 tsp. to c. tandoori spice

2 chicken breast

20 tsp. olive oil

40 cl coconut milk

2 oak leaf

pepper

fleur de sel

Slice the chicken breast into thin segments. Marinate them in the refrigerator for 1-5 hours with the oil, spices, salt, and pepper. Then, roast them in the pan with the marinade for 10 to 15 minutes.

Peel, then rinse and whirl the salad. Mix the coconut milk, coconut flakes, and half of the lemon juice to make the coconut vinaigrette.

Wash the avocados under running water, press them dry, and then cut them in half lengthwise to remove their kernels and skin.

Slice them into segments and add the remaining lemon juice. Begin preparing the dishes with the salad and avocado. Chicken and germinated seeds are sprinkled on top of this dish. Enjoy a coconut sauce seasoning.

The Chicken Pesto, Vegetables, And Fresh Parmesan On The Ketogenic Diet

2 tomato

A sachet of sautéed vegetables

A bowl of cream cheese

600 g chicken

2 tablespoon pesto

Chicken with pesto, vegetables, and grated cheese preparation:

1. Cook the chicken and cover with pesto on both sides.
2. Cook the vegetables.
3. Cut the chicken into pieces, add the vegetables and tomatoes and mix.
4. Add fresh cheese to your taste.

Egg Salad

Ingredients:

2 Avocado, peeled and pitted, then sliced thinly
 4 tablespoons coconut oil
 2 teaspoon thyme
 4 hard-boiled fresh eggs , chopped
Pinch of salt

 4 cups mixed salad greens
 2 red bell pepper, seeded. Slice thinly
 2 green, yellow bell pepper, seeds and thinly sliced 1 cup cherry tomatoes, halved
 2 small cucumber, thinly sliced

fresh eggs Method:

Combine coconut oil, thyme, a sprinkle of salt, and pepper in a bowl.

Combine salad greens, cucumber, tomatoes, bell peppers, and avocado in a large salad bowl.

The salad is tossed with the oil mixture after it is poured over it. The salad is served with minced fresh eggs on top.

Fresh Eggs 6 . Sardine Salad

Ingredients:

8 cups mixed salad greens

4 teaspoons Capers, rinsed
1 Cup Black Olives,

500 g sardines in tomato-based sauce

2 tablespoons apple cider vinegar
4 tablespoons olive oil

chopped:

Whisk olive oil, tomato sauce, and apple cider vinegar together in a basin, then set aside.

In a large basin, combine salad greens, black olives, and capers.

In a basin, combine the sardines and the dressing. Then, carefully combine ingredients.

Serve without delay.

Immediately season with salt and pepper and serve.

Maple Bacon Bulletproof Coffee

Ingredients:

- 2 tsp vanilla extract
- 4 tbsp sans sugar maple syrup
- Whipped cream for topping
- 2 bacon cut, cooked and crumbled

- 2 cup newly prepared coffee
- 2 tbsp MCT oil
- 4 tbsp butter
- 2 tsp maple extract

1. Add every one of the fixings aside from the whipped cream and bacon to a blender, and interaction until

smooth.

Pour the beverage into an enormous glass, twirl a few whipped cream on top and trimming with the bacon. Enjoy!

Shepherd's Pie

Ingredients:

4 lbs. ground beef

2 c bone or veggie broth

4 heads cauliflower

2 c butter

1 lb. bacon, chopped

4 c shredded carrots

4 c diced celery

Directions:

1. Cut and steam the cauliflower.
2.   Put it in a food processor or blender. Add the
3. butter and blend until nice and smooth. Set it aside.

4. Cook the bacon in a large fry pan, and then add the carrots and celery. Continue
5. cooking for about 5-10   minutes while you preheat the oven to 350 degrees F. Add the
6. ground beef to the fry pan along with a little salt and about half the broth.
7. Simmer and stir, adding more broth if it gets dry.
8.   Cook until the broth has

9. evaporated and the beef is cooked through.

10.   Spread the beef mixture in the

11.   bottom of a large baking dish with high sides.

12.   Spoon the cauliflower on top and

13.   smooth.

14.   Bake uncovered for about 60 minutes until top starts to brown.

Sugar-Free Vanilla Bean Ise Cream

Ingredients

• 200 gm Butter, grass fed, unsalted (melted; or ghee)

• 100 gm Cacao butter (melted)

• 120 gm Bulletproof Brain Octane Oil

• 100 gm Coconut oil (melted)

• 4 tbsp Stevia sweetener, powder • 4 tbsp Water, filtered

• 4 tsp Vanilla bean powder

• 8 medium egg Egg (pastured-raised)

• 8 medium egg Egg yolk (pastured-raised)

- 2   tsp Lemon juice (or apple cider vinegar)

Instructions

1. Add all the ingredients into a high-powered blender and blitz for 1-5 minutes.
2. Taste the mixture and adjust the sweetness to your liking.
3. Pour into an ice-cream maker and churn for 35 to 40 minutes.
4. Serve and enjoy this incredibly nourishing and delicious ice-cream.

Fried Fresh Eggs With Spinach

8.

Ingredients:

4 cloves garlic, minced
4 red onions, diced
1 teaspoon dried oregano Pinch of salt,
pinch of pepper

12 fresh eggs
1000 grams ground beef
4 cups spinach
4 tablespoons coconut oil

Method:

1. Trim spinach, then coarsely mince before setting aside.
2. In a large skillet, sauté onion and garlic in heated coconut oil until golden.
3. Add oregano to the skillet and thoroughly combine the ingredients.
4. The mélange is seasoned with salt and pepper.
5. Add the minced beef to the pan and continue cooking for approximately 5 to 10 minutes.
6. Cook the spinach for an additional 1-5 minutes, or until it has wilted.
7. Add freshly beaten eggs to the mixture, stir, and continue cooking

for approximately 1-5 minutes, or until the eggs are set.

8. Transfer fresh scrambled eggs to a plate and serve immediately.

Sweet Potato Ginger Brownies

Ingredients:

1 tsp. ground ginger

½ tsp. vanilla powder

½ tsp. baking powder

pinch sea salt

1 c chopped Lindt 90% dark chocolate bar

4 c cooked mashed sweet potato

6 eggs

½ c butter

½ c raw honey

6 T coconut flour

6 T dark cocoa powder

4 tsp. ground cinnamon

Directions:

1. Preheat oven to 350 degrees F. Mix the mashed sweet potato with the eggs,

2. butter, honey, and vanilla. Combine well.

3. Add in the coconut flour, cocoa powder,

4. spices, baking powder, and salt.

5. Again mix well. Stir in the chocolate pieces.

6. Spread the batter in a buttered 8x8 pan. Bake 70 to 80   minutes until a toothpick

7. comes out fairly clean. Cool before cutting.

Salmon And Zucchini Grilled

2 pound zucchini, cut into 1 -inch slices

4 tablespoons plus 4 teaspoons Bulletproof Brain Octane oil 2 teaspoons minced fresh oregano

8 tablespoons fresh lemon juice

8 teaspoons high-quality olive oil

Sea salt

4 skin-on wild salmon fillets skin scored lightly

8 teaspoons finely chopped fresh herbs

Heat a grill pan over (or fire up your grill to) medium-high heat.

In a medium bowl, toss the zucchini with 4 tablespoons of the Brain

Ostane oil. 6 to 8 minutes, or until the zusshni is fork-tender, grill the zusshni over a low flame or heat, turning the zusshni midway through. Set the grill to run ade (or leave it on). To taste, season the zucchini with oregano, 2 teaspoons of the lemon juice, olive oil, and sea salt. Set aside.

If using a grill pan, preheat it over moderate heat. Rub the salmon with the remaining 2 tablespoons of Braian

Ostane oil and then sprinkle with sea salt. Place the salmon on the grill grate, skin-side down, and cook for approximately 6 minutes, reducing the heat to medium-low as necessary to prevent the skin from charring. Approximately 36 minutes longer, flip the fillet with care and continue cooking until the salmon is medium-rare.

Add herbs and the remaining 2 tablespoons of lemon juice to the fish. Season with sea salt and serve alongside the zucchini.

Classic Eggs Benedict With Bulletproof Fresh Eggs

Ingredients:

-Dash of Sea Salt For Taste

-4 Fresh eggs , Softly Poached

-Some Hollandaise Sauce

-2 Tbsp. of Butter, Unsalted and Grass Fed

-2 Avocado, Ripe

-6 Handfuls of Spinach, Washed and Drained

Directions:

1. Using a medium sized pan, add in your spinach
2. with about 4 Tbsp. of Water. Sauté your spinach until slightly wilted.
3. Then strain the water from your pan and add in your butter and salt.
4. Continue to sauté until the butter is fully melted.
5. Place your spinach onto a serving plate.
6. Place your poached fresh eggs on top of your spinach and drizzle with a touch of hollandaise sauce.
7. Serve with a slice of fresh avocado and enjoy.

Stuffing Morning Beef Patties

Ingredients:

-2 Tbsp. of Thyme, Fresh and Organic

-2 Tbsp. of Rosemary, Fresh and Organic

-2 Tbsp. of Coconut Oil, Organic and Extra Virgin

-4 Pounds of Beef, Ground and Grass Fed

-2 tsp. of Sea Salt For Taste

Directions:

1. Preheat the oven to 350 degrees Fahrenheit.
2. Then, in a large mixing basin, combine the beef with the freshly ground herbs and a pinch of sea salt.
3. Using your hands, thoroughly combine the ingredients until thoroughly combined.
4. Then, shape the mixture into dense patties.
5. Then, lubricate a medium-sized baking pan with coconut oil and cook the patties for the next 25-30 minutes, or until they are fully cooked.

Fennel & Citrus Side Salad

Ingredients

½ cup flat leaf parsley, chopped

Juice of 2 lemon

6 tablespoon virgin olive oil

Salt and pepper to taste

4 fennel bulbs, finely sliced

2 tangerine, segmented

Method

1. Combine all the ingredients together in a bowl.
2. Serve immediately.

Avocado Filled With Garlic Shrimp

Ingredients

2 clove garlic, minced

Juice of half a lemon

½ cup parsley, chopped

Salt and pepper to taste

4 large avocados, stoned

1 cup wild caught tiger prawns, raw

½ cup grass fed butter

Method

1. Bring a small saucepan to a medium heat.

2. Add the butter.
3. When the butter is melted add the garlic and prawns. Mix well.
4. Cook for around 5 to 10 minutes or until prawns are cooked.
5. Stir in the parsley, lemon and salt & pepper.
6. Fill the avocado with the prawn mixture, enjoy!

Cauliflower Curry

Ingredients:

½ cup water

2 teaspoon curry powder

4 tablespoons cashews, chopped

2 head cauliflower

2 cup coconut milk

Method:

Rinse cauliflower with water and pat dry. Trim and separate the cauliflower florets.

Place the cauliflower florets, cashews, coconut milk, and water in a saucepan and sauté over medium heat for approximately 1-5 minutes.

Remove the pan from the heat and mash the cauliflower with a spatula.

Before serving, season it with curry and a sprinkle of salt.

Spiced Spaghetti Squash

Ingredients

2 tablespoon coconut oil

2 teaspoon cumin

1 teaspoon turmeric

2 tablespoon parsley

2 large spaghetti squash

2 tsp coriander

1 teaspoon salt

1/2   teaspoon cayenne

Directions

1. Using a sharp knife, delicately pierce the squash multiple times to prevent it from exploding in the microwave.
2. Microwave on high for approximately 1-5 minutes, turning halfway through.
3. Allow the squash to chill enough to be handled before slicing it lengthwise.
4. Utilize a fork to remove and discard the seeds.
5. The interior should be scraped into a medium basin.
6. Blend and shred the fibers until they are finely separated.
7. Stir in the coriander, salt, coconut oil, cayenne pepper, turmeric, and cumin to the spaghetti squash.
8. Be sure to thoroughly combine them before serving.

9. Serve warm with parsley sprigs on top.

Paleo Coconut Nectarine Smoothie

Ingredients

2 tablespoon ghee or grass-fed

5 cups peeled, diced sweet potato

2 teaspoon of fresh oregano leaves

Sea salt

2 teaspoon fresh thyme leaves

2 cup low-sodium chicken broth

2 tablespoon coconut or MCT oil

5 cups peeled, diced butternut squash

Directions

1. In a medium saucepan containing oil, melt the ghee over medium-low heat. If using leek, add it and simmer for one minute, stirring frequently and taking care not to let it brown. Stir the herbs, squash, and sweet potato once to combine.
2. Add the broth and salt to the bowl. Simmer gradually and stir occasionally for approximately 35 to 40 minutes, or until the squash is just tender and the sweet potato is soft.
3. If desired, taste and add more salt as desired. Serve hot.

Rack Of Lamb With Roasted Vegetables

2 Tbsp. Rosemary

2 Tbsp. Ground Turmeric

Salt

4 C. Fennel, Sliced

4 C. Celery, Sliced

4 C. Cauliflower, Sliced

2 Tbsp. Ghee

2 Rack of Lamb

2 Tbsp. Sage

2 Tbsp. Thyme

Preheat the oven to 350 degrees Fahrenheit.

Spread the ghee on the rib of lamb. Add salt and minced herbs.

Place the vegetables in a roasting pan and the lamb on top of the vegetables with the fat side facing down.

Bake for approximately 45 minutes.

Turn the broiler on low and broil the skin side up for a few minutes to brown it.

Smoked Salmon And Fresh Eggs

Ingredient List:

•   8 Tablespoons of Ghee, Grass Fed Variety and Fully Melted

•   2 teaspoon of Dill, Fresh

•   Dash of Salt, For Taste

•   8 Fresh eggs , Pastured Variety and Poached

•   1 Cup of Salmon, Smoked Variety and Wild Caught Variety

Instructions:

In a large skillet set over medium heat, melt the ghee first. Once the ghee has completely dissolved, add the dill and cook for at least thirty-six seconds. Turn off the furnace.

Divide the smoked salmon between two serving dishes. Finished with poached eggsFresh eggs and stewed dill are combined in this dish.

Season with a pinch of salt and serve immediately. Enjoy.

Carrot Variation

Ingredients:

12 celery sticks including tops, chopped into chunks

4 large carrots, topped, tailed and chopped into chunks

20 asparagus spears, chopped into chunks

Method:

1. Push ingredients into juicer.

2. Make sure to alternate ingredients as they being pushed into the juicer so the mixture is an even consistency.

Cauliflower Combo

Ingredients:

1 small head cauliflower, broken into pieces

1 tsp turmeric powder

8 large carrots, topped, tailed and chopped into chunks

Method:

1. Push ingredients into juicer.

2. Make sure to alternate ingredients as they being pushed into the juicer so the mixture is an even consistency.

Salad Of Spinach And Cranberries

- 1-5 tablespoons water

- 4 tablespoons organic almonds slivers

- <u>2   1 tablespoons organic extra virgin coconut oil</u>

- 4 cups organic kale, finely chopped

- 6 cups organic spinach

- ½ cup dried organic cranberries

1. Heat coconut oil in a frying pan.
2. Take care that it does not get overheated.

3. Add in chopped kale with a tablespoon of water.

4. Kale has to be softened which would take about 5 to 10 minutes of cooking.

5. Once kale looks done, throw in the cranberries and again cook for 5-10 minutes.

6. Finally add spinach and cook it till it turns limp.

7. Toss in almond slivers and turn off the heat.
8. Always remember that if you are using kale or spinach in a recipe, it should always be cooked.
9. This is a very simple recipe gets ready in a jiffy and takes only about 20 minutes to prepare for 5 to 10 people.

Grapefruit Smoothie

Ingredients:

- 10 drops stevia
- 2 tablespoon upgraded XCT oil
- 2 0 ice cubes
- 1 cup pink grapefruit, sliced and chopped
- 6 celery stalks, chopped

- 2 tablespoon grass-fed butter
- 2 cup coconut milk, unsweetened

Directions:

1. Place ice cubes into a food processor.
2. Add remaining ingredients in order and process for 1-5 minutes or until blended.
3. Serve immediately.

Banana Radish Smoothie

Ingredients:

- 4 radishes, washed, sliced
- 4 tablespoons grass-fed ghee
- 2 tablespoon upgraded collagen
- 1 cup unsweetened coconut milk
- 2 medium banana
- ½ cup ice

Directions:

1. Place ice cubes into a food blender.
2. Add banana and radishes.
3. Process until smooth; add remaining ingredients and process until frothy and blended well.
4. Serve immediately.

Vinaigrette That Is Refreshing And Light

Ingredients:

½ cup extra virgin olive oil

4 tablespoons MCT oil

Handful fresh basil, finely chopped

½ cup apple cider vinegar

1 avocado

Preparation:

1. Blend all ingredients in food processor until smooth.
2. Pour over your favorite Bulletproof salad.

Hearty Chicken Soup

Ingredients:

16 cups water, filtered

2 inch fresh ginger, peeled and finely chopped

Sea salt, to taste

2 pound ground chicken, grass-fed and organic

2 cup celery, finely chopped

2 cup broccoli, chopped

2 cup spinach, finely chopped

2 cup cauliflower, chopped

Preparation:

Bring vegetables, water, ginger, and sea salt to a simmer in a large pot. Add additional seasonings, such as thyme or oregano, if desired. When water is boiling, add chicken to the mélange directly. Once the chicken and vegetables are sufficiently cooked, remove from heat and serve.

Bombs Of Broccoli And Cheese

½ of a cup of parmesan cheese, shredded

½ of a cup of Colby jack cheese, shredded

15-20 pieces of broccoli that have been steamed until they are tender

1. Blend the broccoli and cheeses in a blender until they are thoroughly integrated.
2. Ensure they can be shaped and formed into spheres.

3. Form them into small spheres and compact them by pressing them together.
4. Heat a deep fryer or pan with at least 1-5 an inch of vegetable oil and place the explosives in it so that they become crispy.
5. If using the pan method, flip at least once.

Salami Pickle Rollups

½ of a cup of cream cheese

2 glass jar of small dill pickles

12 slices of salami

Spread your cream cheese evenly across the salami segments. Place the pickle on its side in the middle and wrap it up. The cream cheese should help it adhere, but you may need to use a toothpick to keep it rolled up while transporting it to work or eating it. Additionally, you can slice the parts into piwheels.